The Fat Ass Guide to Losing Weight
Tony Xhudo, M.S., H.N.
Board Certified by A.A.D.P.

The Fat Ass Guide to Losing Weight
Tony Xhudo, M.S., H.N.
Board Certified by A.A.D.P.
Published by Dawn Xhudo
Copyright 2012 Dawn Xhudo

DISCLAIMER

DISCLAIMER: This information was gathered from sources including textbooks, and reports. Neither the author nor publisher assumes any liability for the information presented in this text. This book is not intended to provide medical advice. The purpose of this reference book is only to provide a compendium of information for the reader, for entertainment purposes only. Readers should consult with appropriate medical authorities before using any related products and the proper legal authorities if unsure of the status of substances described herein.

DISCLOSURE

Tony Xhudo M.S., H.N. ALSO THE AUTHOR OF:

How to Build Muscle in Your Advanced Years

The Ultimate Guide to Enhancing Your Sex Life

The Everyday Guy's Guide to getting & having More Sex

Smart Nutrients for Smart Babies

The Secrets of gaining Mass Muscle Made Easy

The Anabolic Edge to Mass Muscle

Ergogenic Aids for Bodybuilding

How to Build Muscle The No Nonsense Way

The Woman's Guide to Burning Fat and Building Muscle

Ergogenic Aides for Bodybuilding

How to Lower Cholesterol Without Drugs

Holistic Therapy For Fibromyalgia & Chronic Fatigue: The Cause & Remedy

Aphrodisiacs: Proven Sex Boosters That Work

Old School Bodybuilding: Training With The Legends

The Everyday Guys Guide to Getting & Having More Sex

TONY ALSO IS THE AUTHOR OF:

Muscle Health & Fitness Blog:
http://musclehealtandfitness.blog.com

Gaining Mass Muscle:
http://tonyxhudo.wordpress.com/

TABLE OF CONTENTS

INTRODUCTION
THE FAT ASS GUIDE TO LOSING WEIGHT

After 35 years in the field of health and fitness, I've seen so many of my clients and people suffer needlessly from obesity, with the multitude of implications that stem from it like heart disease, high blood pressure, depression, diabetes, liver disease, high cholesterol and list seems to go on forever. I witnessed the disparity of how their diets did not work and how it affected their lives. Many believed that their lives were ruined, devoid of being happy in leading a product-ed life. Obesity is a serious illness that we need to pay attention to, affecting so many young children and adults. As a concerned holistic health practitioner, my priority and concern lies with the general public in educating the general public about health and well-being.

With so many available books on weight loss and planned diets, it's a wonder that no one can lose the weight they hope to lose. In the battle against fat, only the smart ones achieve what most of us only long for, permanent weight-loss. The National Weight Control Registry (NWCR) that was created in 1993 by researchers at Brown Unversity and the University of Colorado, states that 95% of dieters that lose weight, gain it back. Diet companies make a great deal of money advertising quick weight loss idea's and gimmicks. Doctor's preach eat a healthy diet and exercise, Nutritionists tell you to plan a structured diet according to your metabolism. Personal trainer's tell us they can do it through personal training and exercise to burn off the excess calories. So, who do we believe?

Well, actually they kind of are all right in what they preach and some are wrong, so here we go again. But I'm here to tell you that there is a way to lose all the weight your heart desires. I am not selling anything like a quick weight loss plan or gimmick. Neither will I say that there is a secret in weight loss that has been kept from the public for along time now, nor will I say that there's some magical formula either. What I'm trying to say here as a concerned health practitioner, its really not that complicated a matter. Its actually so very simple that you probably have known this all along but found it out to be too easy and simple, and its true, it is very easy to lose all the weight you possibly could want to lose.

That is why I wrote this short book to inform you of the correct and easy way to lose weight. But before we do, I would like to explain to you the how's and why's of weight-loss. We are going to discover how by reading this book we can prove the weight loss industry wrong in their money making schemes on weight-loss that actually never go away, but returns back with a vengeance. Weight loss is a very lucrative money making proposition for all those involved. Diet supplements, weight-loss meal plans sold in grocery stores, nutritionists, and weight loss centers all make tons of money on your grief of being obese. As long as there's obesity, and people are desperate to lose the weight, there will always will be a market for it.

No different then anything else, it's always about the money and not for the concern of health and well being. By the time you have read this book you will know all there is to know about how to eliminate hunger pangs, cravings, and fat-loss. The main focus of this book is to lose weight and enhance your well being and to keep the weight off that you lost for good.

<u>CHAPTER 1</u>
IT'S NOT YOUR FAULT

Well, its not your fault that you've gained all this weight, blame the Federal Government for allowing all the food commercials on television that advertise food products that offer no nutritional value, except empty calories of fat. Blame the FDA for also allowing the food industry for lacing the foods with excess sugar and salt, and trans fatty acids. Know that Sugar and salt are our bodies two primary ingredients that affect our satiety levels. They know that the human's brain primary fuel is glucose (sugar). So they set every one up by pumping heavy amounts of sugar into their products, like soft drinks, juices, cakes, candy, pastries, and even condiments like mustard, salad dressing, ketchup America's favorite condiment.

One table spoon equals 17 grams of sugar, wow ! 17 grams too much, and people then often wonder why we carve certain foods and condiments so much. We as concerned people and parents that have children must be knowledgeable in what we are putting into our stomach. People need to really start reading the ingredients on the labels that are put there for our convenience, but how many people often read labels? Well not that many I can tell you. Here is a brief list for you're information just to see what you're missing and consuming, and then we wonder why our children are obese, and then say things like, I don't know where he or she get that, obesity does not run in my family , nor does it in my husband's.

- **Ketchup = 17grams of sugar per tablespoon.**
- **1,000 Island Salad dressing = 2 tablespoons of sugar.**
- **Honey Barbeque sauce = 36 grams of sugar**
- **Sweet Pickle Relish = 1 tablespoon 15 grams of sugar**
- **Prego Marinara Spaghetti Sauce = 1 serving ½ a cup 120 grams of sugar**

<u>The average American consumes 150lbs of sugar per year.</u> Many health experts and scientists state that sugar is toxic and should be regulated. It might taste good, but sugar is very addictive and is fueling the obesity epidemic. The obesity epidemic is just getting worse with each year that passes, and those who are concerned are looking for answers.

Sugar is addicting just as much as narcotics, alcohol, and other controlled substances are, and the food industry knows this. So when they add fructose to their products we often buy more. That is why its just about found in everything.

Know that there are 5 tastes on your tongue, sweet, sour, bitter, salty, and hummie, and sugar covers up the taste of the other 4, so you can not taste the the negative aspects of foods. You can even make dog poop taste good if you add enough sugar in it, and in essence that is what our food industry has done. The question is how much more metabolic syndrome and diabetes do we need to see before we even consider to change the policy of fructose regulation in foods?

We as Americans are the fattest people in the world today with one of the highest cases of diabetes in the world. Why? Because of Sugar !

 - *"If we the people let the government decide on what foods we should eat and what medicines should we take, our bodies will soon be in a sorry state as the souls who live in Tyranny"- The Late Thomas Jefferson*

If you ask me, I personally do not think that our government actually cares about what we eat, all they care about is how much we can spend ! Then why as we, a great super power have the worst health care system's in the world today. It's because disease's boil down to making money. There's no money in cure's for illnesses, the money is in the medicine that helps to keep us alive just long enough for us to keep on spending, yes my friends, I've studied holistic medicine long enough to know that cure's can be found for illness and life threatening disease's, but lets be realistic and realize the whole picture here. Remember, the money is in the medicine and not the cure. This is the same thing concerning weight loss. Have you every asked yourself why do we as Americans have the most obese people on the plant today ? Because of greedy politicians and lobbyist's that exploit our people to create disease and illness for the sake of the American dollar, that's why!

Sickness for those in the industry is big money. Think about it, if our government really cared about health care and the American people, there would less ad's about pharmaceutical drugs and junk foods laced with tons of sugar and salt advertised on t.v. And newspapers and magazines. Instead, if they preached healthy foods and educated more people on proper health care and eating the proper diet and eliminating sugar products then there would be less needs for us to make doctor appointments. In the 1940's there were less than 10% of the American population that were considered fat or obese. Today over 80% of the people in America are obese or their on their way in becoming obese, and yet obesity is still getting worse year by year.

Why are we also considered the fattest people on the plant ? I wonder if its anything to do with fast food restaurants like Mc Donald's, Burger King, Kentucky Fried Chicken, Taco Bell, Wendy's, etc. Is it because we are lazy or maybe that the food just tastes so good and is convenient?

CHAPTER 2
READ THE LABELS

The alternate names for sugar and forms of added sugar are: corn syrup, high fructose corn syrup, dextrose, fruit juice concentrate, lactose, maltose, malt syrup, molasses, cane juice, cane syrup, and sucrose. Be aware of any ingredient ending in "ose" is likely sugar.

To find the sugar hidden in your everyday foods, read the nutritional facts label and the ingredient list carefully. There is also differentiation between naturally occurring sugars and added sugars on the label. Keep in mind that if the product has no fruit or milk in the ingredients, all of the sugars in the food are from added sugars. So says the American Heart Association. Manufactures often add different kind of sugars during the canning or packaging process, which adds more calories to the food without any nutritional value at all. Knowing what foods have added sugar can help you make healthier food choices and reduce your over all sugar intake.

By law companies must disclose how many grams of sugar a product has in each serving. Look for additives like forms of sugar listed above as an ingredient, then you've found your sugar. Even if it says zero grams. In an ingredient list, items that are more prevalent fall first. With any of these in the first three or four ingredients, you now know you have a major problem. Sweeteners usually fall first after flour and grains. High fructose corn syrup often falls third in many common foods, sodas and fruit juices. Learning to read the labels can go a long way in helping you and your family avoid all the common health problems that hidden sugars create.

Obesity opens up a whole new door to a posse full of killer diseases that plague us today like heart disease, strokes, diabetes, and respiratory problems. Its no wonder the World Health Organization states that obesity is the dominant global issue we are facing. Today they are over 61% of Americans that are over weight and facing health issue's that are diet related. In the average American diet sugar has become a mainstay as a source of energy. How did this happen and why did it happen. We would think that our government would take notice on some sort of prevention on the wide spread issue's that sugar has created. A simple fact that you should know how such large companies as Coco Cola and Pepsi switched from a 50/50 mixture of corn syrup and cane sugar to 100% high fructose corn syrup, enabling them to save over 20% costs, and boost portion sizes and still make a profit.

There is a new science of understanding human satisfaction or satiety, and the evidence seems to show that there is no actual thing as satiety. Between 1970 and 1994, the individual food intake in America increased by 200 calories more per person. By 1999 heavy users of fast food ate more than 20 times per month accounting for profits in the fast food industry of 66 billion dollars of 110 billion dollars spent on fast food. The great innovation here in America is the "freedom to order in" and 40% of the average American's food budget is spent on takeaways. Fat consumption also doubled between 1977 and 1995, from 19% of calories to 38%.

The American national dish isn't Thanksgiving Turkey or Mom's home made Apple Pie, but a toxic mixture of sugar and more sugar, and Coco Cola and Pepsi. Statistics do show that American's are eating more and more, and the caloric intake has gone up drastically in the last four decades. Over weight and obesity has risen to huge proportions that make us the fattest country in the world. But there are things that we can do, and that is why I chose to write this book.

WEIGHT-LOSS METHODS THAT WORK

There are so many methods that one can use to lose weight, such as weight loss programs, fad diets, various pills, weight-loss drugs, hypnosis, and many exercise programs that claim to be successful. As with each of these methods, one can find testimonials claiming how much weight they lost. But they never tell you how much weight they gained back after months of being back on their regular routine. That's the problem, long term results is what is the most important fact here. Most of these weight loss methods work on a short term solution. Meaning in the long run your weight returns back with a vengeance.

Getting someone to follow a planned diet is one of the most difficult things to do, why? Because we're creature's of habit. Everyone is basically set in their own eating habits. Dieting is one of the most simplest forms of weight control, and definitely one of the most common. Because going on a diet seems extremely logical and people gain weight because they simply eat a lot of foods, especially the wrong foods. It makes sense that was the reason how they got heavy in the first place. So to lose weight you do the opposite and stop eating, but not completely of course. Its just a matter of knowing what to eat. There are certain foods that do speed up the metabolism and there some that just provide heavy calories that only create fat reservoirs in the body.

Like I said earlier, dieting is extremely hard for most people simply because they have trained themselves indirectly to eat a certain way that has become a hindrance to themselves. Why ? Because we tend to eat what is convenient and taste good. So for that matter it becomes a challenge for many to follow certain diets. There are some people that can adhere to it and which most can not. Its not a surprise that most people that do go on a diet simply give up before the results start flowing. The stress of dieting and counting calories become too much for them to bare.

The majority of diets can be divided into 3 groups: low carb diets, low fat diets, and calorie restriction diets. What scientists really say about the effects of these types of diets on weight loss is that it does not really matter which one you go for. There is also one study that says low-fat diets are no more effective than other types of diets. Most people typically like low carbohydrate diets because they lose more weight the first week than on other type of diet. But this brings us back to what I've said earlier because the weight loss in this case was only temporary due to the elimination of body water that was retained.

Calorie restriction diets are one of the most frustrating ones because people have to spend most of their time counting calories, which is not always easy to do. The real truth here is diets are an effective weight-loss method if they are planned sensibly. If you are not eating a certain type of diet due to a health problem, then you can basically eat anything within moderation. You just have to cut down on un-healthy foods and replace them with healthy ones. Recent research shows that effective weight loss doesn't revolve around the amount of calories coming from protein, carbohydrates, and fat. The newest studies and research from the Institute of of Medicine, Food, and Nutrition Board show that there are wide ranges of each of these nutrients.

You can choose to eat high protein, low protein, low carbohydrate or high carbohydrate, low fat or high fat. Because in terms of long-term weight-loss it really does not matter. The only type of diet that does work for long-term results is caloric restriction. The percentages of calories from protein, carbs, and fats does matter in other aspects of health, but not in weight-loss. Calorie restriction diets is one of the few things that is proven to prolong longevity. By limiting the amount of food you consume, you'll not only slow down your aging process, but you'll also help prevent and avoid heart problems, diabetes, and a host of others. The calorie restriction movement is getting a lot of press and attention from the longevity movement.

Unlike typical diets that focus primarily on weight-loss, calorie restriction is about reducing long term caloric intake and by consuming adequate nutrients at the same time in the pursuit of a more energetic lifestyle. There numerous studies that show by eating less foods can help you live a longer and healthier life. By cutting calories, which eventually lead to weight loss and a slower metabolic rate, can lengthen the human life span. While there is no specific meal plan to follow, you generally eat 20% to 30% less than what you would normally consume or is recommended. Sugar and saturated fats, and most dairy products are not recommended. While vegetables, fruits, and grains providing most of your calories.

Know that the people who do lose a significant amount of weight and keep it off do two things; they restrict the amount of calories they eat, and they exercise for a half hour or more each day.

THE HEALTH BENEFITS ASSOCIATED WITH CALORIC RESTRICTION AND EXERCISE ARE:

- **Reduction in blood pressure**
- **Reduction in heart rate**
- **Improved LDL Levels**
- **Reduced Triyglycerides**
- **Reduced body fat levels**
- **Increase in lean muscle mass**
- **Insulin sensitivity**
- **Improved blood glucose levels**
- **Reduced free radical damage from oxidative stress**
- **Improved HDL Levels**

To lose weight easily cut back on your caloric intake, reduce your portion size of your meals. Stop snacking on junk foods, eliminate processed foods, and the worst – stop drinking all soda's. Know that each can of soda is equivalent to 12 teaspoons of sugar. Start using meal replacement shakes as a meal substitute, researchers in Spain discovered that there was a big difference in weight-loss in those people that substituted a meal replacement drink for a meal. They also concluded that a low calorie meal replacement was an effective weight-loss aid.

The key to weight-loss is cutting calories through dieting than through exercising. But for most people its probably more difficult to eliminate the amount of calories through exercise than you can do through dieting. That is why cutting calories through dieting is generally more effective for weight-loss than exercising. But by doing both, you can gain a very big advantage in weight-loss. Just remember that exercise can speed up the burning effect of weight-loss even further.

There are approximately 3,500 calories in a pound of stored body fat. So if you create a 3,500 caloric deficit through diet, exercise or a combination of both, you will then lose one pound of body weight. This combination of diet and exercise has been proven best for an effective long-term weight-loss result.

If you want to lose fat, a very useful guide for lowering your caloric intake is to reduce your calories by 500, but not more than 1,000 calories below your maintenance level. As a guide to minimum caloric intake, the American College Sports Medicine recommends that calories never drop below 1,200 calories per day for women and 1,800 calories per day for men.

An alternative way of calculating a safe minimum caloric intake level is by reference to your current body weight. Reducing calories by 15% - 20% below your daily caloric maintenance needs is a useful start, in which you can also increase this depending on your weight-loss goals.

Please do not be fooled by all these infomercials that promise these "they don't want you to know" secret formulas and quick weight-loss schemes. Because there is no secret magic pills or an exotic potion of any kind. Like I've mentioned before, the weight-loss industry is a very large lucrative business that want to make a quick buck and get rich off of your money and hard work.

It never surprises me with the many ad's and infomercials that state their secret ingredients in their effective weight-loss products will make you lose weight while you sleep. With all the many diet programs, weight-loss supplements, and you name it, then why are we American's leading the whole world in obesity ? If they all actually did work. Big pharmaceutical drug companies make billions of dollars on our hard earned money advertising and selling their weight-loss drugs. Now we have the "HCG Diet" consisting of human chorionic gonadotropin injections dirived from pregnant Woman's urine. But in actuality HCG was used by a British doctor Albert T. Simeons, contending that HCG injections could enable dieters to live on 500 calorie diet a day. However, later on scientific studies demonstrated that wasn't the case and that the given injections of HCG didn't seem to cause any weight-loss.

To this day HCG does not seem to be an effective weight-loss aid in the treatment of obesity and there is also no substantial evidence that it can increase weight-loss beyond that resulting from calorie restricting diets. Please, do not be fooled by these gimmicks that offer no scientific proof or backing at all. There is no secret cure for obesity and no, they don't use pregnant woman's urine (HCG) as injections for weight-loss, and that goes for the homeopathic versions as well. The real reason why people can lose weight is caloric restriction and exercise.

FOODS & SUPPLEMENTS THAT MIMIC GOOD EFFECTS OF CALORIC RESTRICTION

If you can not develop enough will power or self control to limit yourself away from caloric intake, there are products or supplements that will help a great deal in helping you manage caloric restriction. Scientists have found out that there are a variety of herb's and foods, that have a great potential to help you limit your caloric restricted diet. Some of these herb's work on the brain's satiety level by limiting your cravings and hunger pangs by affecting your brain's Serotonin levels. More on that topic later.

I believe that with the use of calorie mimic agents in conjunction with a calorie restricted diet is central to long term weight-loss that you will be able to keep off permanently. The combined use of these caloric mimicking supplements can go a long way when combined with some form of exercise.

NATURAL FOODS & SUPPLEMENTS TO HELP LIMIT YOUR CALORIC CONSUMPTION

1. **Avocados – increases insulin sensitivity and rich in essential fatty acids with vitamins & minerals.**

2. **Resveratrol – potent anti-oxidant & anti-aging benefits.**

3. **Carnosine – inhibits glycolazation from sugar which produces metabolic syndrome and type 2 diabetes.**

4. **Acetyl-L-Carnitine – facilitates mitochondrial function.**

5. **Gymnema Sylvestra – helps with blood sugar balance and metabolism.**

6. **Cinnamon – acts like a natural insulin.**

7. **Green Tea – increases the livers ability to burn fat.**

8. **Ellgagic Acid – potent anti-cancer agent.**

9. **Alpha Lipoic Acid – potent insulin sensitizer and powerful anti-oxidant.**

10. **Leptin – stimulates fat metabolism.**

11. **Chromium – regulates blood sugar balance and increases insulin sensitivity.**

12. **Vandium – modulates blood sugar balance.**

13. **Maritime Bark Extract – anti-cancer and potent anti-oxidant.**

DRUGS USED

1. **Metaform – anti-diabetic drug that enhances insulin sensitivity.**

2. **Thiazoladinediones – anti-diabetic drug that enhances insulin sensitivity.**

Bare in mind that the use of these caloric mimicking supplements should be used in the context of a healthy diet with meaningful limitations on total caloric intake. These nutrients have shown to generate many of the same effects in the body as caloric restriction, with out significant changes to dietary modifications. Take it slowly when cutting calories by 500 calories per day. When trying to lose weight, most experts recommend in losing 1 to 2 pounds per week as a safe realistic weight-loss goal. Still while most of us can benefit from modest calorie cut backs while incorporating mostly whole grains, fruits, vegetables, lean meats, beans, and low-fat dairy foods in our diet. Combing that type of a diet with exercise, a proven disease fighter, can help you achieve a healthier body weight, preserve muscle and bone, and give you a big psychological boost.

CHAPTER 3
EXERCISING & WEIGHT-LOSS

To lose weight one needs to burn more calories than they take in. Even light walking is a form of exercise and for those that don't want to spend time in sweaty gym's, you can increase the intensity by doing power walking with some 2 to 5lbs dumbbells swinging your arms back and forward simultaneously, which will increase the effectiveness of the exercise. For those more physically challenged, you can do cardio on a treadmill, stair master, or do a full body workout. Whatever suits your needs or desire. The point is to include some form of exercise to speed up your metabolism, and combining it with a calorie restricted diet to get the best of both worlds in your quest for weight-loss.

For walking, you can start out slowly for a walk around the block and then eventually increase it two blocks and so forth. Try and not worry too much about your body weight, the most important thing to do is be concerned about your health and how you are going to establish a proper and healthy diet that is going to sustain you in your calorie restriction program. The rest will come easy as you go along with the help of the caloric mimicking supplements which will benefit you that much more efficiently. When you can start to burn about 3,000 calories per week at a moderate and intense level of activity, you will then begin to see improvements in every health care marker that exists like blood pressure, cholesterol levels, triglycerides, and body-fat composition.

No matter what form of exercise you should choose, you will begin to see improvements in over a weeks time and still be able to improve as the weeks progress even further. You will begin to feel your health improve in so many facets that you will be proud of like, sleeping habits will improve, your sex life, and even if you have diabetes type two, the exercise will cure it. The number of calories burned through exercise varies according to the type of exercise and the weight of the person. Typically moderate exercise can burn approximately 300 calories per hour. In general people that exercise also have a lower death rate than those who do not, regardless of their weight. Exercise is important during the initial implementation of a calorie restricted program, as it has been found that bone density is reduced by weight loss induced by calorie restriction, but not by exercise-induced weight-loss.

IMPORTANT EXERCISE TIP'S

In order to improve body composition, you must increase muscle and lose fat. Know that muscle weighs more than fat. When you gain muscle you lose fat, you may weigh more according to the scales. So let the mirror be scale not the judge. Having more muscle also speeds up your metabolism, you will be able to burn more fat. The best way to triple your fat loss efforts, is to combine strength training with cardio training for the best possible results. When a high intense strength training routine is combined with cardio training, you triple your effects of fat-loss. An important fact to consider is to target the amount of stomach fat around your belly which has been an indicator to cardiovascular disease and diabetes.

Its also important to add specific abdominal exercises if that is the case pertaining to you. Start by adding aerobic forms of exercise in the beginning or Pilates to just get you motivated enough, to later target it much more specifically. The bottom line on exercising is to think of it in a long term scenario as of something that will benefit you for the rest of your life. Exercise does not have to be burdensome, it can be something as light as power walking, aerobics, or cardio, or you can go at all out and include some weightlifting training. Find the motivation that you need and get going and prove to yourself that you can look and be fit just as well as others are, and be proud of yourself and your achievements in weight-loss.

ADDITIONAL METHODS THAT HELP WITH WEIGHT-LOSS

We have already discussed how caloric restriction and exercise stimulate permanent fat loss, however there are some other methods that do help in weight loss that we will begin to explore in this chapter. With weight loss being the most talked about hobby in America today, why ? Because we all care how good we look in clothes, swim suits, and to be just generally happy and healthy.

HOW DID WE BECOME SO FAT?

With so many fast food eateries and food establishments in just about every street corner or mall in America, its kind of hard to resist the aroma of a hamburger or steak brewing in the air. Sometimes we just can not seem to help ourselves, after all we're just human and we do have our weaknesses. With each passing year, more American people either eat out in restaurants or order in for food. Then its back to T.V. Time on the couch with our remote in our hand and bowl of dip and chips nearby to snack on. Let's not forget our cola's or Pepsi to wash it down with. That's how easy we as Americans get to start on our way of obesity.

This sort of thing, food binging goes on just about in every house in America, and its no wonder why we're the fattest country in the world. We have no else to blame but ourselves, for watching infomercials on T.V. about all the delicious snacks that bring on cravings, so then off to the refrigerator we go.

CHAPTER 4
FOOD ADDICTIONS & CRAVINGS

These bad eating habits that we tend to develop over time start to become second nature and now we have a food addiction problem. This goes back to what I was saying earlier about sugar and salt, the two primary cravings and main ingredients that are added to so many foods in this country. Large food manufactures know this and they do spike a large amount of foods in the grocery store shelves. All of your can goods and anything in a box has either sugar or salt. How many times have you had the urge or craving for a piece of chocolate or potato chips or even a box of Krispy Kremes?

These food cravings are not a sign of weakness on your part, but a change in your brain's chemistry involving your brain's levels of serotonin, our brain's feel good chemical. Most often, the foods we crave are processed carbohydrates that affect the brains level of serotonin. People with food addiction problems may symptoms like headaches, mood changes, insomnia, irritability and depression. They often can relieve these symptoms temporarily by eating the foods they crave. Also, people with food cravings may actually have neurochemical and hormonal imbalances that trigger these cravings. If you think that you may be serotonin deficient and want to increase your serotonin levels without resorting to a pint of chocolate ice cream, trying these alternatives may help to eliminate some of your cravings and hunger pangs:

1. Avoid stimulates like caffienated drinks, cigarettes, and amphetamines.
2. Get 60 minutes of moderate or moderately intense exercise on a daily basis.
3. Avoid alcohol.
4. Eliminate any suspected food allergies, paying special attention to gluten(wheat, rye,oats)
5. Make sure your getting a good nights sleep.
6. Certain supplements like 5-HTP (5-hydroxytryptophan) that can help you balance your serotonin levels.
7. St.John's Wort is another serotonin enhancer that will balance moods and cravings.
8. Vitamin B6 – a B vitamin that is needed by the brain in the metabolism of serotonin.
9. SAMe – (S-adenosyl-L-methionine) also helps to balance serotonin and the brain's neurotransmitters.

I believe with the use of these caloric mimicking agents in conjunction with a calorie restricted diet is central to long term weight loss that you will be able to keep off permanently. The combined use of these dietary calorie mimicking supplements can go along way when combined with some form of exercise. These nutrients have been shown to generate many of the same effects in the body as caloric restriction with significant changes to dietary modifications.

Physical cravings may also be a result of low-fat intake or low blood sugar problem. A piece of fruit, yogurt or a handful of nuts can get the blood sugar levels back up and keep you from reaching the unhealthy snacks we think that we may be craving. Emotion also plays a big part in food cravings. When we are stressed out, anxious, frustrated and lonely, can also trigger you into bingeing on snacks. Food addiction can become a dependance no different than a drug addiction can, acting as a coping mechanism. How many of you, have turned to food when bored ? I know I have !

It sort of takes the place in your mind of having something to do and kind of makes you feel calm, doesn't it ? There are pleasure centers in the brain that certain foods stimulate, and the food manufactures know this and do take advantage of this by spiking foods with sugar or salt. No different than smoking cigarettes which affect your brains dopamine system, a neurotransmitter that governs out pleasure center in the brain. Dopamine is our feel good chemical that is also responsible for many of the addiction problems that we suffer today, from gambling, drug use(cocaine), smoking, and food cravings.

So here's the dilemma, unlike people who have problems with drugs or alcohol, people who over eat excessively, and can not give up food entirely are slowly killing themselves in the form of obesity, diabetes, high blood pressure and cardiovascular disease. But there is a solution, eat foods that are nutrient dense that are sustaining and give you health and strength. Every week try and introduce something healthy as vegetables, that you do not normally eat, a fruit that you normally do not buy like kiwi's, blue berries, grapes, straw berries, and natural whole foods that your body can assimilate and process that will be better for you in the long run. Every week try and introduce nuts, whole grains, oatmeal, fresh fish, vegetables of all kind. This will help you break the habit and dependance on processed and junk foods. If cravings do take over, have a piece of celery or carrots, or a piece of fruit.

There are also food addiction work shops that might be of help for those that have trouble or lack the will power in succumbing to their addictions. Food groups like the "Food Addicts Anonymous" can be found online for the nearest one near you. It should be pointed out that there are different varieties of food addiction. For instance, there is compulsive over eating, where the individual goes on eating binges for several days. Symptoms include eating quickly, compulsively eating alone, and eating when there is no evidence of hunger. Yet another form of addiction is bulimia, in which the individual over eats, then purges either by vomiting or by taking laxatives. Signs of this addiction includes isolating one's self from when eating, trying to consume huge portions of food rapidly, and being preoccupied with one's weight.

Food addicts often follow the tenets of the same kind of 12 step program used by alcoholics. This involves admitting the powerlessness over food, their belief that their sanity could be restored, and an admission of their faults and failings. Below is a list of symptoms associated with food addictions:

- Disorders including bulimia, compulsive eating, and anorexia are all characteristic of food addictions. Food addicts also gain an immense pleasure anticipating, and making food available.

- Food addicts are obsessed with the amount of food they eat, their body image and their weight.

- Secretive eating is a common sign. A food addict isolates themselves and gobbles everything up from the fridge.

- Eating bad and wrong foods is another sign. Eating food that is raw and under cooked, stale, and eating junk foods, sweets or even bread compulsively.

- Food addicts eat to relieve stress and worry.

- They eat often till they get sick.

- A feeling of anxiety while over eating is exhibited, and a feeling of guilt when they over eat remains.

- They also often eat very fast so they can eat some more.

- They eat everything on their plate even when they are full.

A 2006 study published in the "Lancet" revealed that eating fast food increased the risk of developing type 2 diabetes. Another study in 2009 at the University of Minnesota, revealed that children who watch T.V. For more than 5 hours a day are more prone to become fast food junkies as adults, which was determined by researchers to be the cause of watching too many fast-food related commercials on television. Here's a scary fact, today's children in America may actually have a shorter life span than those of their parents. The simple fact behind this is, we always tend to over eat the wrong type of foods. Often a particular craving may point to something lacking in your diet. ***Here is a list of particular cravings and what it may point to:***

DECODING YOUR FOOD CRAVINGS

<u>Chocolate</u> cravings – A Magnesium and Copper deficiency. Take a vitamin/mineral supplement with your meals and eat more raw nuts, seeds, and legumes and fruits.

<u>Fried foods</u> – Calcium & Omega 3 fatty acids deficiency. Try eating more deep water ocean fish like tuna, mackerel, halibut, and sardines.

<u>Salt craving</u> – Hydration(drink more water), B Complex, and Chloride. Could be also be the

result of poor adrenal gland functioning. Start salting your foods with natural sea salt which contains true sodium and iodine. That's why most people often will crave bags of potato chips. Regular table salt contains absolutely no benefit at all.

<u>Sugar cravings</u> – Craving sweets throughout most of the day could be the result of an under-active thyroid problem. Eat more fish and use sea salt with your foods, a natural iodine source and vital minerals that's great for an under active thyroid condition.

<u>Dairy Product cravings</u> - Calcium deficiency.

<u>Carbohydrates</u> - First thing that is reached for when stressed from over racked nerves. Liquid magnesium and B complex vitamins will negate this problem.

<u>Sweet & Sour cravings</u> – Your liver is trying to cleanse itself from impurities.

<u>Dirt cravings</u> – You would be surprised how people out there actually have had a dirt craving. It actually means your deficient in trace minerals. Purchase a good vitamin mineral supplement rich in trace minerals.

<u>Spicy Foods</u> – Thyroid imbalance or also a sulfur deficiency, Eat more raw garlic and horse radish.

<u>Caffeine</u> – this relates to an exhausted adrenal glands. Use licorice root extract, vitamin B5, B complex, and vitamin C.

<u>Nicotine cravings</u> – Often relates to emotional issues, Dopamine related, B complex deficiency, and tyrosine deficiency.

<u>Alcohol cravings</u> – (alcoholism genetically related) severe vitamin B1 & B2, and the amino acid L-Glutamine.

<u>Ice cravings</u> – Iron deficiency. Eat more lean red meats, poultry, fish, seaweed, greens, and black cherries.

<u>Beets</u> – Iron deficiency.
<u>Meat cravings</u> – Could be the result of constant thinking which make for the craving of protein and its amino acids to replenish brain function. Amino acids and mineral deficiency, especially phosphorus.

<u>Bread & Toast</u> – This is a nitrogen deficiency, eat more protein foods, lean meats, turkey, chicken, or drink a 100%whey protein shake.

<u>Burned Foods</u> – A carbon deficiency. Eat fresh fruits.

<u>Cool Drinks</u> – A Manganese deficiency, eat more walnuts, almonds, pecans, pine apples, and blue berries.

<u>Oily Snacks & Fatty Foods</u> - A Calcium deficiency, eat mustard greens, turnip greens, broccoli, kale, cheese, and legumes.

Pre-Menstrual cravings – A Zinc deficiency, eat more lean red meats, especially organ meats(liver, kidney, heart), sea food, leafy vegetables, and all root vegetables.

Foods that are high in fat and sugar assist in the production of serotonin, the neurotransmitter that helps us feel calm and relaxed. So when we eat the same foods we crave, we remember that it worked and we may return back to that same food the next time we need a fix. Behind every craving there's a nutritional deficiency. Your body craves specific foods, because it needs specific nutrients that can be found in that particular food. So, most people don't know what nutrient they are actually craving and reach out for the worst possible choice in "filling the void." That is why after eating a bag of chips you still crave salt and after eating an entire box of brownies, you still want more. This phenomena is known as "false cravings." next time you have a craving for that particular food like something sweet, salty, or spicy, think about what your body is really carving for. So try taking or eating something that is full of nutrients instead, to something which corresponds to the list above on cravings and what they nutritionally mean.

Cravings do definitely have a physical component in which they give some insight into what type of person we are. Doctor Alan R. Hirsch, head of the Smell and Taste Research Foundation in Chicago and author of "What Flavor is Your Personality" that has studied more than 18,000 people for over 25 years states that when you crave salt, you may have a mineral deficiency. Studies reveal that people who eat a low-calcium diet want more salty food. One reason is, Sodium temporarily increases calcium levels in the blood, which tricks the body into thinking the problem is solved. Researchers have also found that there may be a shortage of other minerals too, such as lack of potassium, calcium, and iron which caused test subjects to devour regular table salt. Dr. Hirsch also "describes salt lovers as an external locus of control," meaning that outside forces, not

their own actions, determine their fate. When you carve for something as sweet as chocolate, and what it says about your body is the flavor makes you swoon – it does that because of the release of serotonin. Dr. Hirsch states that its basically a dessert acting as an anti-depressant seeking out a quick lift satisfying your moods. The body absorbs refined sugars of the candy variety faster than any other type of food, giving you an immediate type of fuel. Dr. Hirsch states that sugar fiends tend to walk on the wild side, and describes them as hedonistic, with few regrets. They also like to stand out and feel special.

Spicy food cravings with some people that become addicted to the rush of the fiery taste, the spiked blood pressure, accelerated heart rate, and rapid breathing are people who are having difficulty cooling down, so your body craves a fiery taste to make you perspire.

What that says about you is – you like order in your life, dislike wasting time, and sweat the details. But when your body craves both sweet and salty, your body is in the need of glucose and sodium to function properly. What this says about you – is you may be a loner, private person, creative, a wiz, and to a point standoffish.

As you can now see cravings are normal and almost everyone has them. No one also needs to feel guilty or unusual about having food cravings. Successful weight-loss as it pertains to food cravings may be one of the most important keys in weight control and in the type of foods you crave. The most identifiable thing about foods people crave is that they are highly dense in calories. An alternative to food craving is to substitute foods that taste similar, but have fewer calories, since the craving can be satisfied by related tastes. So by controlling the frequency of giving in to cravings rather than suppressing them, may be an important area in future weight control problems to consider.

Next time your faced with a tantalizing treat that you would rather skip, try this phrase - "I Don't Eat That !" new research finds that 80% of women who used those words stuck with their good eating habits, compared to 10% of the women who said "I Can't." saying I can't means you're giving up something desirable, says study co-author Vanessa Patrick PhD. Associate professor of marketing at the University of Houston. "But by saying I Don't gives you a sense of empowerment." A diet strategy that works.

CHAPTER 5
FOODS YOU MUST STOP EATING TO LOSE WEIGHT

Well you've heard the expression, "you are what you eat." Well, in regards to weight loss, 'what you eat' is almost important as 'how much you eat'. By eating a healthy and well balanced nutritional plan will help you lose weight and keep it off. Most people think they know which foods are healthy and which are not. Example, are salads, I wish I had a dollar for every time I heard someone say 'all I eat are salads'. Most people mistakenly believe that eating salads are healthy, but the salads most people eat cause more weight gain than weight-loss. The reason salads are unhealthy is because of the toppings they put on the salads, like salad dressings a thousand island's, creamy ranch, blue cheese dressing, and french dressing. These dressings are very high in calories and sugar. They should only be used if one is trying to gain weight.

Deli meats that get added in your salad are also a no-no. Bacon and fatty deli meats are also high in fats and calories as well. Topped salads with fried chicken also not a good idea. Also keep the croutons off your salad, you don't need the extra calories. Fatty cheeses can just as well turn a good salad bad. Instead, you should use healthy nut topping's, olive oil or vinegar a an added healthy ingredient.

Beware of foods labeled "fat -free", of all the foods being heavily marketed as "free" of a potentially harmful nutrient, fat-free foods are the worst. These foods are typically full of calories just as much as their full-fat counter-parts. If you eat more than the designated serving size, those fat grams and calories can add up. So, its best to just enjoy a small portion of the whole fat version, which wrecks less havoc on your body than the fat-free version with all its flavor enhancing additives, particularly sugar.

 Re-duced-Fat Peanut Butter is another be aware product, the truth of the matter with regular peanut butter is, there's no real reason to take out the fat. The fat in peanut butter is a combination of polyunsaturated fat and monounsaturated fats which are actually healthy for you, so why take it out ? But when you take out the good fats from peanut butter to make a lighter version, **sugar** is added to replace the flavor and calorie difference is negligible. Which means the reduced fat version does not mean you can eat more than its full-fat counter part. So, its better to stick with the natural version of peanut butter which should just contain peanuts and salt. Peanuts are high in calories and are a healthy choice, so just keep an eye on your servings.

Diet Soda's, for people watching their calories or who have diabetes, diet soda may be a better option than regular soda. However from a nutritional standpoint, there is nothing redeeming about diet soda's, they don't have calories, and they don't have anything that's

good for your diet either. Diet sodas also contain artificial sweeteners to enhance the flavor of the drink, the consumption of artificial sweeteners are known to cause the increased risk of metabolic syndrome, which is a group of metabolic factors that put a person at an increased risk for coronary artery disease, stroke and type 2 diabetes. Look for instead drinks that offers nutrition – even if it has calories and sugar if you must have it, such as orange juice. If you crave the "fizziness" of a soda, try a calorie free seltzer water with a splash of lemon in it. You can also brew a batch of home made unsweetened ice-tea. Just know that what ever you're consuming, to pay attention to what you're consuming, so read the labels.

Frozen yogurt, however is not just the same thing as frozen. Most frozen yogurt sold at the super markets and retail stores have been heat-processed, which kills the beneficial live cultures. Real yogurt contains live, active cultures that keep the good bacteria in your digestive tract healthy. Look for instead low-fat yogurt if you choose to indulge with a small serving. If toppings are desired add fruit slices without added sugar. Stony Field Yogurt, organic has live beneficial cultures that are certified organic.

LIST OF UNHEALTHY FOODS TO AVOID

1. **Soda Pop – Very acidifying and chemically laden, loads of sugar and artificial flavoring**

noted to cause Alzheimer's Disorder. Try and avoid them, instead drink water or make your own juice from a juice machine.

2. Fried Chicken – Laced with farm additive steroids thats covered with gluten rich breading, MSG, salt, and high in calories and fat and chemicals that can make you sick. Instead use organic chicken breasts broiled.

3. Bacon Cheeseburgers – where to begin ? Loaded with fat, hormones, cholesterol, anti-biotics, and calories. Instead opt for a veggie burger with avocados.

4. French Fries - These are simply unhealthy fat salt bombs, fried in rancid oil that often never gets changed. Instead fry your own french fries in coconut oil.

5. Milk Shakes – loaded with saturated fats, sugar, dairy, and chemicals for flavoring. Milk shakes can leave you sluggish and sick. Skip it and have a home made smoothie with fruit and yogurt.

6. Deep Fried Cheese Sticks – Loaded with fat, salt, hormones, and anti-biotics and fried in rancid oils. Skip this and have some veggie sticks.

7. Fish Sticks – unless its whole cold water species of fish

8. Pepperoni Pizza – The cheese and white flour are combined with nitrosamine containing salty processed meats, and is un-healthy made this way. Instead make it yourself with whole natural ingredients if you need to have it.

9. Nachos with Cheese – Corn chips loaded with meat, beans, sauce, cheese and dipped in sour cream, really ? This is a high fat, high calorie death bomb. Instead have some veggie sticks dipped in slasa.

10. Hamburger with Chili – The beef is laden with hormones, anti-biotics, and fast food beef is known to contain E-coli bacteria and some gross ingredients. Instead try a vegetarian chili made with natural ingredients.

11. Hot Dogs – Come from a variety of left-over meat trimmings that include organs of animals that were slaughtered and processed with salt, paste, and other un-healthy chemicals. Plus organ meats are known to contain diseases. Instead try a veggie sandwich.

12. Cheese Cake – No better than fast food sources just listed. Its loaded with salt, sugar, chemicals, and hormones. Try instead chia pudding.

13. Taco's – Beef, chemicals, hormones,anti-biotics, and fried GMO corn which all the ingredients contribute to an un-healthy snack. Instead have a taco salad with black beans and salsa sauce.

14. Beef Burrito – The beef and cheese are the biggest problem that are loaded with anti-biotics, dairy and hormones. Try instead a taco salad or veggie burger.

15. Chicken Nuggets – This is a mainstay of children around the world which is actually terrible for you. Made from mechanically separated chicken parts that's hormone laced with anti-biotics, white flour, salt, sugar, and copious amounts of corn by-products, all of which can harm and destroy your child's health. Instead give them almond butter with celery sticks or carrots as a snack.

16. Cold Cut Sandwiches – The good old American stand-by sandwich that's loaded with preservatives, sodium, nitrates, high fats, and contaminated animal products. Try instead and have a veggie wrap or hummus.

17. Teriyaki Chicken – Believed to be a healthy meal by many people, but in reality is loaded with sugar, sodium, nitrates, MSG and other un-healthy ingredients. Try brown rice with vegetables.

18. Chef's Salad – Consists of eggs, lunch meats, fat laden dressing, salt, sugar, and all the other bad stuff that comes with meat. Instead make yourself your own salad with dark green leafy salad with your home made salad dressing.

UNHEALTHY INGREDIENTS

The result of all this fast food in America has been growing by leaps and bounds, and obesity is on the rise in all age groups from young to old, with youth obesity being the major concern. Disease is also on the rise too, with much of it being attributed to the cause of obesity on a dietary level of junk foods that inflict so many with harmful chemicals laced with foods such as meats laced with hormones and antibiotics to increase the farmer's yield at the farmer's market, and the new chemical additives used for various types of seasoning and flavoring.

Fast foods are the worst bunch of them all, with unhealthy ingredients as fructose corn syrup (HFCS), that can be found in ketchup, mustard, mayo, fries, deserts, salad dressings, and all bread products.

It is no wonder that we as a country have the highest cases of diabetes type1 and 2. Gluten another bread product that comes from wheat flour, is also found in buns, sliced white bread, and other bread products that the human body has a hard time processing. That is why in the industry its called fast food, it's basically a fast way to enter the hospital. Well, you now are well aware of the dangers and concepts of fast foods, junk foods, and of how they cause obesity and other related diseases.

CHAPTER 6
OTHER HELPFUL SUBSTANCES & TIP'S TO LOSE WEIGHT

Weight loss products are such a big commodity that can be found in just about any convenience store, grocery store, drug store's, health food stores, and even gas stations sell some sort of weight loss aid. The shelves are stocked with fat-burners, appetite suppressants, diet-aids, and thyroid simulators. All of them claiming to enhance weight loss to some degree. Most of these commercial products have many of the basic and same ingredients, which can be caffeine, gurana, green tea, chromium (blood sugar balance), theobromine, coleus forskolii, ma huang, cla, l-carnitine, synephrine, and thyroid stimulators.

NATURAL APPETITE SUPPRESSANTS

Natural appetite suppressants are becoming more sought after because people are beginning to realize that some diets are hard to adhere to. They do work and make it more likely for you to be able to come to terms with your planned diet. With planned diets, it may be difficult for those that do have extreme cravings for the wrong food of choice. Below is a list that you will find helpful in search for natural appetite suppressants that can be of help for those who often find it difficult to refrain from their cravings of junk foods and snacks.

1. <u>Hoodia Gordonii</u> – A natural appetite suppressant that is found in South Africa, that has become quite a popular diet aid in the weight-loss market. Hoodia can reduce your hunger pangs, appetite and calories, fooling your brain in thinking that your full. Dosages may vary with individuals, so read the manufacturer's description. Comes in tincture form (liquid) or in capsules.

2. <u>Caralluma Fimbriata</u> – Similar to the effects of Hoodia, that also helps to increase one's stamina. Caralluma is known as a famine food in India that will quench your thirst and curb your appetite. It has gone under extensive studies and clinical trials for reducing hunger and simultaneously reduce belly fat.

3. <u>Tryptophan</u> – An amino acid that gets converted in the brain to the neurotransmitter serotonin. Tryptophan is the main precursor to serotonin that has also be used for a variety of disorders, including appetite control, anxiety, insomnia, eating disorders, and depression. Tryptophan enhances the release of serotonin from neurons in the brain which help with decreasing your appetite levels. When we eat fewer carbohydrates, we tend to lose weight, so by raising serotonin levels we can thus lower our binge eating and control our hunger pangs. Tryptophan can also be taking any time during the day, always on an empty stomach and at bedtime for a sound an effective sleep. Dosages may vary from person to person and it may range from 1,000mgs to 3,000mgs in divided dosages throughout the day.

4. <u>Water</u> – Yes, believe it or not, water can be an effective and healthy aid in helping you to control hunger and weight-loss. Fresh drinking water, 8 oz's every time you feel the urge to binge will find it to suppress your appetite in nearly every case. If you drink a full glass of water and have the discipline to wait 10 minutes, you will find your appetite is either completely gone or dramatically reduced.

5. <u>Vegetable Broth</u> – This will do the trick if water does not seem to help reduce your cravings. Purchase a 32oz quart of natural, organic vegetable broth. The key is to get organic vegetable broth that does not contain excitotoxins, which contain ingredients that cause neurological disorders that over excite and harm nerve cells. Those ingredients are MSG, yeast extract, autolyzed yeast extracts, hydrolyzed vegetable proteins and similar ingredients. You can also choose organic chicken broth as well for the flavor. Drink it like soup and feel full on only 20 calories, and not like getting 1200 calories from a Big Mac sandwich.

6. <u>Green Leafy Vegetables</u> – Lettuce, cabbage, bokchoy and other leafy vegetables, eaten raw or stir fried in olive oil with onions and garlic. You can eat as much as you want and don't even have to worry about counting calories and feel full with nutrious nutrients that will sustain you.

7. <u>Natural Organic Pickles</u> – Read the ingredient label and make sure you are getting organic pickles free from artificial flavoring and coloring. Very low in calories and you can eat as much as you wish making you feel full and healthy.

8. <u>Apples</u> – So true as the saying goes, "an apple a day keeps the doctor away." loaded with health nutrients and fiber that will help you feel full for most of the day. Apples are great

appetite suppressant foods, because of the bulky fiber fill up your stomach and turns off your appetite control hormones before you over eat.

Also remember, you don't want to starve yourself by eating these very low calorie foods and appetite suppressant agents all day long. Starvation is also the fastest way to train your body to hold on to body fat. These are just idea's to help you get through the difficult time periods when your appetite is at its extreme. Keep in mind that weight loss takes effort and patience, and most of all a carefully planned dietary routine, and discipline. I will outline an effective sample strategy for you in the end of the book to help you better understand the methods described in this book.

NATURAL THERMOGENIC AGENTS

If you want to turn the heat in helping your body to burn calories at a faster rate, there are some things that you can do to stimulate a diet induced thermogenesis. Some people can eat huge portions of food without gaining weight, while others gain weight easily. Part of this phenomena is thermongenesis. Body (somatotype) Ectomorph, Endomorph, and Mesomorph are also a contributing factor. The Ectomorph types have a faster metabolism than either the Endomorph or the Mesomorphs and dissipate extra calories through thermogenensis. Over weight and obese individuals typically have a defective thermongenesis mechanisms, particular the Endomorph body type. Metabolism is the problem, which is related to somatotype metabolisms.

Somatotypes

1. **Ectomorphs – Are slim, lean, long bones, thin faces, long lean legs and arms, fast metabolism which prefers light foods – chicken, fish, and veg's. They can eat a lot of food without gaining weight.**

2. **Endomorphs – Round face, round body type, gains weight easily with a slow metabolism. Frequent hunger cravings that crave carbohydrate foods that are usually high glycemic index foods like french fries, potato chips, candy, etc.**

3. **Mesomorphs – Are muscular body types that have thick muscles and bones, add muscle very easily, and have a medium metabolism. They crave meat and proteins.**

Most people are a combination of two somatotypes, and there are many that fit the genetic description of one particular body type. Regardless of body types, the average person desires a minimum of excess body fat. One of the most effective methods in burning fat, is to include thermogenic agents. Thermogenic nutrients can increase the number of calories you burn. This comes as an ideal situation for those who are predisposed to obesity that have a decreased diet-induced thermogenesis even after they have lost weight and become lean. So for those who seem to have a hard time losing weight, thermogenic agents or nutricuticals can really help you to speed up weight loss. Its no wonder that 90% of the dieters have a difficult time in weight loss. As some diets do tend to suppress thermogenesis, which is the opposite in what you need. You want to speed up your metabolism, not slow it down.

Diets that support themogenesis are high protein diets, low calorie diets, low carb diets, very high fat diets, low sodium diets and fasting. The best time to ingest thermogenic agents is half hour before meals. See the list of thermogenic agents that were listed previously in chapter 5.

OTHER NUTRIENTS THAT ACT SYNERGISTICALLY WITH THERMOGENIC AGENTS

1. **Ferulic Acid – found in rice bran.**
2. **Coenzyme Q10 – normally deficient in obese people.**
3. **Magnesium**
4. **Potassium**
5. **Niacin**
6. **B-vitamins.**
7. **Chromium Polynicotate**
8. **Garcina Cambogia**
9. **Ephedrine (illegal in some states)**
10. **Coffee, Tea, cola nut.**
11. **Growth Hormone supplements for GH production.**
12. **L-Arginine (an amino acid) stimulates the production of GH.**

For those people who fall under the percentages and are not genetically blessed in their metabolism, thermogenic agents, utilized safe and effectively can be a great help in speeding up one's metabolism in allowing your body to burn up excess calories and body fat.

THERMOGENIC AGENTS

1. **Green Tea – Science indicates that substances in green tea have thermogenic effects that help to speed up the metabolism and helps to suppress your appetite. Green tea will help in speeding up your weight loss and help improve cardiovascular health.**

2. **African Mango Extract – A great product that helps control your appetite and stimulates weight loss.**

3. **Coleus Forskolii – Has compounds that help to break up fat cells in the body. It also helps to regulate the body's thermogenic response to food bu increasing the body's basal metabolic rate and the utilization of body fat. Make sure you buy the highest percentage extract standardized for at least 10% or more of forsksolii acids.**

4. **7 Keto-Dhea** – Helps to drive liver cells to burn fatty acids for energy. It also stimulates thyroid activity and lowers cholesterol.

5. **Fucoxanthins with Pomegranate Seeds** – Increases the metabolic rate and the rate of fat burning within the body.

6. **Vanadyl Sulphate** – Helps to mimic insulin.
7.

CHAPTER 7
FACTORS THAT SLOW DOWN METABOLISM

Many people that diet in the hopes of weight loss are often frustrate in their results due to under lying factors unknown to them. One of the most common and under lying factor that will decrease your metabolism is an under active thyroid gland. Hypo-thyroid can affect any one at any age or gender. With hypothyroid, your body's thyroid gland does not produce enough thyroid hormone that results in a slow metabolic rate. The thyroid is the third largest endocrine gland in the body, a butterfly shaped gland that is located below the voice box, wrapping itself around the trachia. It is also responsible for producing thyroid hormones essential to such bodily functions as growth, healthy energy levels, and your metabolic rate.

Deficiency of thyroid hormones slows you body's metabolic processes, affecting the regulation of body temperature, contraction of muscle, circulation of blood, digestion of food and elimination of waste. Weight gain and metabolic rate are intimately related. A slow metabolism interferes with your body's ability to burn fat. So those with hypothyroidism often experience weight gain when their condition is not treated properly. This weight gain can lead to obesity, if the underlying thyroid problem is not taken care of. However there are certain nutrients that can help you balance your thyroid along with certain foods that carry the proper nutrients to support thyroid health. Many of the B vitamins, iron, and anti-oxidants all help to counter the metabolic effects of hypothyroidism, and can be found in leafy green vegetables, berries and whole grains. You can also buy certain thyroid supplements as well that will help support your thyroid gland. There are many thyroid formula's that work very well in improving your thyroid function back up to par. Some examples are listed below:

THYROID SUPPLEMENTS TO RESTORE THYROID BALANCE

1. **Thyroid by American Biologics** - A glandular thyroid extract that works very well.

2. **Raw Thyroid Extract by Natural Sources** – Another multi-glandular thyroid extract that works very well.

3. **Thyroid Support by Roex** – A blend of thyroid supporting nutrients that restore the functioning of your thyroid gland.

4. **Amour Thyroid Extract – A premier and popular product that works extremely well. See Amazon.com**

Note: Most of these products can be purchased on line on the internet.

Prescription drugs are another factor that could slow your metabolism down. So can an excess intake of sugar, fat and refined carbohydrates. Not having a enough sleep also negate the affects of a healthy metabolism. Avoid eating foods right before bed time, the body metabolizes food at a slower rate when sleeping which can lead to UN-necessary weight gain. So by just paying attention to these vital factors about your metabolism can have a great influence on your progress to improve your weight-loss in the long run. There are hundreds of thousands if not millions of people that may be unaware of the causes of a slow metabolism, weight loss control, and obesity. <u>The four factors that are prominent amongst people that have a slow metabolism are:</u>

- **The negative effects that stress has on producing excess cortisol that produces body fat and lowers your metabolism. In short, stress can make you fat.**
- **Thyroid problems – people that have hypothyroid are the direct victims that fall under this category.**
- **Candida Albicans – a yeast infection whose toxins produce a slow metabolism along with a host of other problems and symptoms like- Itchy skin, migraines, sinusitis,impaired immune system and chronic fatigue.**
- **Wrong Type of Diet – that is too rich in refined carbohydrates like bread, flour, potatoes, sweets and sugar by-products. Also not consume an adequate water intake.**

CHAPTER 8
ADAPTOGENIC HERBS THAT HELP WITH WEIGHT-LOSS

Stress can make you gain weight, and that has to do with the release of cortisol, your body's primary stress hormone. In today's world its become a way of life for so many people that endure the everyday stress's of life, be what they may, stress is a sign of the body trying to deal with certain difficult situations in life. When we are under stress, the fight or flight response is triggered in our brains leading to the release of various hormones, especially cortisol. Whether we're stressed for what ever reason, our body's respond like we are about to be harmed and need to fight for our lives or run like hell. To answer tis need our body's release a burst of energy, changes in blood flow, and a shift in metabolism occurs.

The problem is, if one remains in this mode or prolonged state in an a amount of time due to chronic stress, your health then becomes of risk. Chronic stress and cortisol can contribute to weight gain, which is why some weight loss products like "cortislim" are marketed under diet aids for weight-loss. Too much stress and cortisol can slow down your ability to lose weight. How many people often binge when their stress's take affect, causing more weight gain due to eating as an out let from stress, there are many that resort to this tactic, binge eating when ever they are stressed. Too much cortisol release causes a shift in your metabolism, making dieting that much more difficult.

People that due experience chronic stress tend to crave more fatty, salty, and sugary foods. These type of foods affect our brain's neurotransmitter levels causing us to think that we satisfied our stress response. The end result in this is UN-necessary weight gain that is stored as body fat. Prolonged stress can also cause changes in your blood sugar levels which often lead to mood swings, fatigue, and conditions called hyperglycemia. Too much stress has also been linked to metabolic syndrome, that can lead to other greater health concerns like heart failure and diabetes. Higher levels of stress even affects how the body stores abdominal fat, which is not only undesirable, but poses greater health risks than fat stored in other areas of the body.

Stress and weight gain are connected in other ways, like emotional eating caused by an increased level of cortisol which can not only make you crave unhealthy food, but cause you to eat more than you usually would. Many experts in weight-loss believe that one of the big reasons we're seeing more cases of obesity in our society in these days is that people are too stressed and busy to make dinner at home. Often deciding to get fast food at the nearest drive thru instead. With all of the demands placed on yourself, exercise may be one of the best things to consider on your to do list. Why ? Cause exercise is a great stress relief mechanism and besides it helps you to counter your weight loss as well. Exercise along with certain herbal adaptogens can help you a great deal in dealing with the every day stress's of life. There are various substances that have been discovered by scientists to help improve your metabolism and stress response. These natural substances are called "Adaptogens" which were originally discovered and tested in Russia.

These adaptogens work in favor of the body and are accepted by your cells, without causing any side effects and yet are very effective in what they do. Part of Russia's success in the Olympic games were due to adaptogens. The term 'adaptogens' was created by Russian scientists to describe a group of natural substances that have certain special qualities. Which consistent of certain substances that help the human body adapt to conditions of internal and external stress. They also help the body resist situations of stress that would normally have a negative impact on its functioning. Adaptogenic herbs are not like stimulants that raise the blood pressure or cause you to feel jittery such as excess caffeine, or like a strong espresso cup of coffee, or guarana and ephedrine. Adaptogens help to restore balance in the body due to un-for seen circumstances that pertain to a stress response.

Adaptogens, for example can help to raise your blood pressure if its extremely low or lower it if its high. Adaptogens tend to stabilize other areas of the body that are not functioning as they should. They are bi-directional because they work in opposite directions depending on whats needed. They can speed up body systems that are slow, like your metabolism, and slow down your system if it is extremely hyper. They can even balance your emotional levels if you are depressed or agitated. Adaptogens can regulate your body's chemistry system in the necessary direction to restore balance.

The adaptogens that are of interest to us are the ones that have affects of improving our metabolism and whose qualities contribute to burning fat, controlling stress, increasing energy, and physical resistance. Below you will find the adaptogens that are of the most interest to your needs:

Adaptogenic Herb's

1. <u>Rhodiola Rosea</u> – **Is an extraordinary herb that was once considered a Russian military secret by the soviet regime. This plants qualities have been the object of extensive studies by research scientists in many other counties besides Russia. The Chinese called "golden root or artic root" and considered it an excellent source of well-being and enhanced sexual performance. The use of this plant has also been documented in old Chinese texts, where it was used to fight all sources of illness.**

   The Russian studies showed it to have an increased therapeutic and curative activity. Even in high doses it did not pose any threats to the human body. Rhodiola increases the body's response to stressful conditions, illnesses, and emotional well being. The main effects of Rhodiola that may interest us is its proven qualities to fight obesity and depression. These results have been proven by Russian research scientists on a large amount of subjects that were involved with the studies. Today there have been a vast amount of American psychiatrists that have started using Rhodiola for the treatment of depression and the avoidance of obesity, unlike any other medication that is often prescribed by doctors for depression that actually cause one to gain weight.

   Rhodiola has the ability of activating the enzyme lipase, which is an enzyme used in the body to break up accumulated fat cells. A big plus is even without exercising, taking Rhodiola increases the break up of fat by 10% , and if you combined Rhodiola with some sort of exercise, the amount of fat you lose increases up an incredible 70% or more. How can you go wrong with an herb that does all of the following just listed. There are further studies that state Rhodiola to be an affective sexual aid for those that have all sort of sexual problems, from impotency, lack of desire, premature ejaculation, erectile dysfunction and infertility. But one of its most important benefits that it offers is its control on cortisol, the stress hormone which was discussed earlier. Rhodiola has the affect of lowering cortisol production and help those who do have trouble slimming down due to the affects of excess cortisol release.
   Rhodiola also has other various effects that deserve mentioning on its affect on metabolism and a few other bodily functions and illnesses. <u>Some of these are:</u>

*Anti-arrythmic effect on the stabilization of heart beat.

*Anti-Stress response.
*Anti-fatigue.
*Anti-depressant.
*Burns body fat.
*Increases energy levels.
*Promotes emotional calmness and stability.
*Anti-anxiety capabilities.
*Improves memory and sexual function.
*Detoxifies the liver.
*Improves mental concentration.
*Improves your learning ability.

Another beneficial fact is its ability to improve your sleeping ability, in that it can help you sleep soundly. As people with high levels of cortisol suffer from insomnia or poor sleeping habits.

Rhodiola also has the ability of controlling cortisol and reducing the production of cortisol if the levels get to be too high. These qualities that Rhodiola has exhibited on the human body make it to be one of the most important adaptogens that we have as a safe and natural product that we can use to better our health without the unnecessary side effects that prescription medications offer. Rhodiola Rosea has been a valuable aid to many people that have suffered from a slow metabolism that has affected their results in weight loss. This is one important herb to keep in mind to help you cope with the everyday stresses that we may endure in life.

1. <u>Ashwaganda</u> – Is a herb that comes from India. In controlled human studies, ashwaganda has been showed to lower cortisol levels by 26%. In one other study, ashwaganda helped to control glucose levels in diabetics much better than prescription medications did. Ashwaganda can help you lower high glucose levels that makes fat, and people that were using this herb also stated that they slept much better and suffered less fatigue. In terms of boosting the body's metabolism, ashwaganda offers you its ability in helping the thyroid gland to function properly. It has the ability to help in the conversion of T4(thyroxine) which is produced by your thyroid into the more active T3 hormone, which is the one that increases your metabolism. There has also been many people that have used ashwaganda for their hypothyroidism that notice a substantial improvement in their energy levels. Ashwaganda helps to speed up your metabolism and helps to prevent stagnation of your metabolism from occurring, which is from the result of T4 converting into T3.

   But one of its most significant qualities is its ability to counter act anxiety levels ranging from extreme to normal levels of anxiety, and its often compared to the medication Xanax in its affect. This calming affect that ashwaganda exhibits is also used to treat depression as well. It has also been used in the treatment of Parkinson's disorder and Alzhiemers disorder as well. Ashwaganda has a wide spectrum of healing that it is often referred to as the Indian ginseng. Its qualities range from an anti-bacterial, anti-fungal, anti-tumor, anti-nervous system enhancer, and as a natural aid to combat a slow metabolism by improving thyroid health and functioning.

2. <u>Guggul</u> – Was used in India to fight obesity. It does this by stimulating the thyroid gland in its production of thyroid hormones, which helps with the production of T4 and T3. When guggul improves the production of thyroid hormones it decreases cholesterol levels as well. Guggul also decreases triglyceride levels. Guggul is an affective way in correcting a slow metabolism, that may have been slowed down due to a diet.

3. Shilajit – Also goes under the name (mooymi) – according to traditional Indian medicine that states "There is no curable disease in the universe that can not be cured by Shilajit", a blackish-brown substance that grows in the high mountain regions of India, Tibet, Nepal, China, Russia, Afganistan, Bhutan, and Kasmir. Most studies have shown Shilajit to be better than the prescription drug "Metformin" at reducing blood sugar problems and even in the reduction of cholesterol. In Russia it has been used to enhance athletic performance. Shilajit has also been known to reduce anxiety and bring calmness to the nervous system. Today it's use's are more of a performance and mild anabolic in which it helps the body by giving it an enhanced recovery from strenuous activity. The effects of Shilajit are accumulative and it should be cycled for a period of 4 weeks on and 1 week off for its greater effect.

Adaptogens are extremely well suited to be used to enhance physical and emotional well being and to prevent disease associated with stress. Today in many other parts of the world adaptogens have become a way of life for some. Countering the effects of every day stress, adaptogens have helped many in seeking relief from high stressful situations and make one better able in coping with one's life situations. Adaptogens help us to modulate our response to stress on a physical level, emotional level, and in an environmental level, and helps to regulate the interconnected neuroendocrine and immune system function. In particular the adrenal function of the body that counteracts the adverse effects of cortisol.

The important thing to remember is that adaptogens help to create homeostasis during chronic stress by regulating the body's adaptive reactions. Maintaining homeostasis also contributes to the proper regulations of biorhythms and circadian rhythms within the body. Including the normalization of body temperature and the production of the hormone cortisol. This ability to enhance the overall resistance of the body is key to their health promoting qualities. When used along with other therapies, they can help to positively alter the course of many acute and chronic diseases.

This important quality that adaptogens share is, its ability to slow down the biological clock of aging, by reducing the impact of physiological aging factors which are stress and oxidation. Maintaining balance is part of life and, as such, is what we knowingly or unknowingly strive for, in the betterment of a healthy, productive and disease free life. Adaptogens can make that difference in our life. I have listed several of the best adaptogens you can find to help you make a better choice.

CHAPTER 9
WEIGHT-LOSS TIPS

Fiber and Weight-loss: Fiber can help with weight-loss because it enhances the sense of fullness, and influences the hormones that regulate food intake. Tufts research illustrates that people who consume an additional 14 grams of fiber cut their caloric intake by 10%, and those that added 12 grams lost a pound per month. Foods that can speed up the weight-loss process or any foods that are high in fiber like, vegetables, flax seeds, and nuts. Most of the people already know that by consuming fiber, it will lead to better health. Its also important to understand how fiber promotes a healthy digestive tract, which is one of the most influential links to excellent health, and without it your intestines have no way of cleaning themselves and staying healthy. Fiber also known as "roughage" helps to clean out any food debris from previous meals, and helps to also prevent "diverticulitis" from your intestinal walls, which result from impaction of food debris that often tends to build up from eating the wrong foods.

Think of fiber as some sort of roto-rooter that flushes out food particles that tends to adhere to the intestinal walls from periodic eating, eventually this builds up and strains the intestinal walls till the intestines blow up with little pockets of impacted food debris. With out fiber in your diet, you then run the risk of getting diverticulitis. There are two forms of fiber, soluble and insoluble fiber. Insoluble fiber moves through the body rather quickly, and it comes from whole flax seeds and vegetables. Consider insoluble fiber as some sort of brush that gently scrubs bacteria from the walls of your intestinal tract and helps to push out waste products and toxins from the body. Soluble fiber is found in fruits, veggies, nuts, seeds, oats and beans. Think of it as a sponge that soaks up excess cholesterol, toxins, and bad bacteria keeping it out from your blood stream. Soluble fiber has been proven to reduce high cholesterol and heart disease risk.

Fiber also helps in weight-loss by stimulating the metabolism. When introducing yourself to a fiber diet make sure that you do not take in large amounts without drinking sufficient amounts of water, as constipation can set in. Increase your fiber intake by 3-5 grams per week and make sure you drink at least 8 glasses a day until your urine becomes clear. Remember if you increase your fiber intake without increasing your water intake, constipation will surely follow. **Below is a list of fiber recommended foods that are high in fiber:**

- **Cauliflower, broccoli, brussel sprouts, and cabbage.**
- **Eggplants, zucchini, and rice.**
- **Flax seeds, almonds, avocado's, and psyllium husks.**

Fruits filled with fiber are :

- **Apples** – regardless of which type, apples are high in fiber and low in calories. Eating apples can make you feel full and will satisfy your hunger.
- **Apricots** – especially rich in insoluble fiber, they absorb more water and will make you feel full and very nutritious for you.
- **Blackberries** – high in fiber and relatively low in sugar.
- **Raspberries** – are low in calories high in fiber. 3 grams of fiber in each cup.
- **Mangoes** – are ripe in fiber and rich in nutrients.
- **Kiwifruit** – high in fiber and low in calories.
- **Dates** – are fat and cholesterol free, and full of soluble and insoluble fiber. Dates help to suppress the appetite.

Fiber is found primarily in carbohydrate rich foods, which is a reason that we need to include a balanced amount of healthy carbohydrates daily. Fiber also helps to keep our bowl movements regular and wards off disease by removing toxins from our intestines, binding them and moving them through our colon that much more quickly to where your bowl movements will become regular.

One of the main reasons we are to include fiber in our diet isn't just for weight-loss purposes, but to also help provide a healthy intestinal function and decreasing disease like high cholesterol, cancer, and heart disease. In general though concerning weight-loss, people who eat a diet high in fiber are less likely to grab a sugary snack for a quick energy fix. So by adding more fiber to your diet, you will likely cause your body to lose more weight and improve your health, but remember to add it slowly to your diet on a gradual level. As rapid increases in fiber will tend to cause intestinal gas and discomfort. Also with out consuming enough water, you can cause constipation instead of helping to eliminate it.

Water consumption and weight-loss: Studies have shown that drinking more water before each meal has been shown to help promote weight-loss. Drinking two 8 ounce glasses of water before meals helps to melt the pounds away. Researchers in Germany report that water consumption increases the rate at which people burn calories. After drinking 17 ounces of water a day, metabolic rate of people increased by30% for both men and women. We need water for our metabolic processes especially if you start to consume extra fiber. There are many reasons for you to drink water, especially if you are dieting. Water assists in digestion, waste excretion, circulation and even in breathing. Dehydration can lead to sugar cravings, fatigue, and irritability. Dehydration also slows down weight-loss by significantly lowering your metabolism.

Drinking ice water allows your body to burn more calories. Compared to room temperature water, ice cold water can burn an additional 10 calories which may not seem like a lot, but in a months time it can add up. Know that the process of burning calories requires an adequate supply of water in order to function efficiently. Do not worry about drinking too much water and it giving you that bloated look. There are a number of causes of water retention, including consuming too much salt. But drinking water is not one of them. Water for your body is like oil to your car, you must consume at least 8 glasses per day to keep your body and metabolism operating efficiently.

LEPTIN: THE KEY TO WEIGHT-LOSS

Leptin, a new comer to weight loss that wasn't discovered till 1994, that has become one of the most interesting hormones for anyone trying to lose weight. Leptin, may also be one of the reasons people often fail in keeping the weight off from following previous diets. Leptin is an important hormone in regulating one's body weight. Leptin is also synthesized and secreted primarily by the adipocytes (fat cells) that is present in the blood stream in direct proportion to the amount of adipose (fat) tissue and as fat cells become enlarged in obesity, they secrete more Leptin.

Did you ever wonder why it was easier to gain weight compared to losing weight ? Leptin signals the brain to regulate the metabolism in order to store or burn more fat. Leptin may very well be one of the most important hormones of the body, because of its wide interest and conditions of the human body. Its receptors are present in tissue's throughout the body, suggesting that it can have a direct effects on other aspects of health. Research shows that 85% of people who have lost weight, ended up in gaining it back, because of the body's metabolic thermostat, Leptin is reset upward automatically. When people lose weight, the production of Leptin decreases, which causes people to regain the weight they had once lost. Leptin being derived from fat cells, which when you lose weight, Leptin levels drop, and when you gain fat, Leptin levels rise. When Leptin levels drop you get hungry, when you feel full from eating too much food, Leptin then go up.

As being affected by by both levels, under eating and over eating, Leptin levels will rise and fall as a direct result of eating habits. Leptin has also been referred to as the anti-obesity hormone, but is now called the ant-starvation hormone, because it tells the brain what to do when our fat levels are in low supply. You would also think it would be desirable to increase Leptin levels, however, in most over weight people, Leptin levels are actually excessively high due to Leptin resistance, a process similar to the concept of insulin resistance.

In today's society food surrounds us and over eating is common. This disrupts the hormonal signals in our body. Eventually Leptin receptors becomes desensitized to leptins affects. Once a person becomes Leptin resistance, the body has a difficult time transporting Leptin past the blood barrier to the hypothalamus where it is needed to send satiety signals. Even though blood levels of Leptin may be excessively high, brain levels are insufficiently low, thus resulting in food cravings and weight gain. Which the brain believes the body is in a famished state and tells it to continuously store fat.

Leptin levels tend to rise as we age, and may be one of the reasons 30 year olds have a less difficult time losing weight gained, then people who are in their 40's and beyond. Further more in regards to women and estrogen deficiency, is related to a rise in Leptin, offering a potential explanation for why women gain weight more easily after menopause. Leptin is also a powerful appetite suppressant, and we even have Leptin taste buds on our tongues which help to regulate the cravings for sweet food. Leptin levels are also excessively high in obese people and this Leptin resistance is associated with weight gain. When you become Leptin resistant, Leptin receptors throughout the body, including those on your taste buds and in the brain, aren't getting the message that food consumption should be stopped. Research indicates that by lowering leptin levels in over weight people can restore this malfunctioning Leptin system and trigger weight-loss.

The primary functional role of Leptin is to defend, not reduce, body fat by increasing appetite and decrease energy expenditure when fat stores are low. Unfortunately there is no easy route of just taking a Leptin pill to help resolve our weight gaining problems. Leptin can't be taken orally, because our stomachs can not absorb it. It would need to be injected for it to be absorbed in every day life for life. A more practical way and healthy solution would be to follow a diet of cycling your caloric and carbohydrate intake throughout the course of a week. A day of controlled over eating will help you raise leptin levels and can help you avoid some metabolic adaptations natural with any type of restricted caloric diet. Sufficient sleep is one of the most important factors in controlling leptin. Like melatonin, Leptin is secreted in the highest amounts at night time, and those with deprived sleep levels will affect the secretion peak of Leptin which will occur earlier disrupting hormonal profiles and encouraging weight gain.

Avoiding sugar and bad fats and instituting a daily exercise routine can also help to a certain extent. There are also some nutritional strategies that one can employ in controlling Leptin levels, to achieve weight loss. Scientists have explored the possibility that a number of nutritional supplements can reduce levels of this weight reducing hormone. As mentioned earlier, *melatonin* plays a key role in regulating leptin levels in the body. Both of these hormones, *melatonin* and leptin work together to regulate body mass and energy balance. A number of studies do show that *melatonin* supplements can lower leptin levels and that the pineal gland helps to control leptin release.

***L-carnitine* is another nutrient shown to induce some promising leptin lowering effects.** After *carnitine* supplementation leptin levels were shown to be reduced by 6%. ***Conjugated linoleic acid (CLA)* has exerted both weight-lowering and leptin lowering affects.** In rodent study, compared to controlled, *CLA* significantly reduced serum leptin concentration by 42% while also decreasing the weight of visceral adipose tissue. *CLA* supplementation produced a 5.2% decrease in body weight compared with the control even though food intake was similar in both groups. Another supplement with leptin lowering properties is _**Omega 3 fatty acids**_. Eating fish may alter the influence of leptin on body fat and help the body become more finely tuned to the signals of leptin sends to the body.

Leptin is emerging as a hormone that is integral to weight management. Studies suggest that the key to successful permanent weight loss, may be the lowering of this hormone. A number of supplements have been highlighted in this chapter, _**Melatonin, CLA, L-carnitine, and Omega 3 fatty acids**_, **all seem to play an important part in the control and regulation of leptin.**

Protein can improve Leptins sensitivity, which lowers caloric intake by helping you feel full faster. Choose quality proteins, like fish, turkey, salmon, lean meats, natural peanut butter, and eggs. You can make a great whey protein smoothie in the morning as a great Leptin stabilizer. The mineral zinc also increases Leptin levels, so include more oysters in your diet, as they have the most zinc per serving. Try and also keep caffeine levels to 1-2 cups a day as it can lower your Leptin levels if consumed in excess. A high sugar consumption can also cause Leptin resistance, especially a high fructose corn syrup as an ingredient. Soda, or candy and anything else with this added ingredient can cause Leptin resistance. Simple carbohydrates slow down the movement of Leptin across the blood brain barrier, so reduce simple carbohydrates from your diet that include white rice, white bread products, cereals, baked goods, and sugar.

CHAPTER 10
LOSING FAT AND KEEPING IT OFF PERMANTLY

There are no supplements or drugs that will make you lose weight and keep it off permanently. To do this you must reduce your caloric restriction per, your body type – ectomorph, mesomorphs, and endomorphs and eat a carefully planned healthy diet with the guide lines laid out in this book and to include a daily exercise program. Know that also pharmaceutical drugs contain side effects that can harm you. A healthy rate of weight loss is to reduce your diet by 500 calories a day by eating nutrient dense healthy foods with added fiber included, and a sufficient amount of water consumed on a daily basis.

A caloric reduction of 500 calories with the addition of exercise can help you lose 1-2 pounds a week. Try and make sure that when adding fiber to your diet to include both forms of fiber, soluble and insoluble and make sure you consume the proper amount of water per day with the addition of the fiber intake. Losing a small amount of weight per week is normal and healthy. Try also to exercise several times per week even if its a light form of walking, whatever may be comfortable for you. You can start out slowly with some light walking or cardio done for 20 minutes to a half hour, then you can advance to some sort of resistance exercise with a planned weightlifting routine. This will most definitely speed up the weight loss.

Join a Food Anonymous Group for psychological counseling that may help curb your appetite control. Approach a proper lifestyle habit towards reducing your weight by eating correctly and by avoiding fast foods and processed foods, and the occasional binge eating at night time before bed time. Learn to also control your insulin levels by staying away from simple carbohydrates and use the necessary supplements to help balance any blood sugar problems that you may have. Also pay attention to a more healthy food intake that will improve your digestive system when eating meals throughout the day. Try and include some more live enzymatic foods by consuming a good balance of foods high in natural enzymes, like pineapples, papaya, and natural organic yogurt rich in beneficial cultures. As great health and a great immune system begins in the stomach area.

Know your food allergies have you have any and learn to avoid them as it can upset and slow down your metabolism and your weight loss results, or see your nearest health practitioner for further advice. Know also that metabolic syndrome is the major cause of obesity and the primary reason in insulin resistance. Reduce your carbohydrate intake and include a bit more quality protein and essential fatty acids like omega 3's, flax seed oil, salmon, and tuna fish, or fish oils. Remember the bigger your belly area with fat induced carbohydrates, the worst off your metabolic syndrome is. Stay away from hydrogenated fats, and sugar by products as the fat cells store more sugar as fat. Avoid artificial sweeteners at all costs, as the have become one of the leading causes of Alzheimer's disease.

Stay away from bad fats as they tend to clog the arteries which include:
- **hydrogeneated fats,margerine, fats from fast foods, trans fatty acids, and fast fats from restaurants.**
- **Good fats to include are – olive oil, natural organic butter, flax seed oil, fish and krill oil, avocados, and nuts and seeds like walnuts. Almonds, pecans, macadamia nuts, sun flower seeds, flax seeds, and pumpkin seeds.**

CHAPTER 11
BALANCING OUT WEIGHT-LOSS – SUMMARY

Everything starts out in the stomach - "we are what we eat" period ! We eat bad, we feel and look bad. So, eliminate all processed foods and take a multi-enzyme with your foods. Do not over eat – but reduce your calories by 500 calories a day, starting out slowly with an included exercise program that will help you lose a health 1-2 pounds per week.

A healthy diet and exercise are the key to long lasting weight-loss. Try and reverse insulin resistance with a proper diet and recommended supplements. Do not crash diet. Make sure you avoid junk foods and eat a nutrient dense meal provided in you diet plan. Always start out your day with a healthy low calorie breakfast. Reduce any stress from your daily activity, use the guide on adaptogens to help.

Join a Food Addiction Group Anonymous if you need help with further counseling on appetite control, or see guide on adaptogens that can help a great deal. Use fish oil supplements with high EPA and DHA levels, or add fish in your diet to get the recommended supply of omega 3 fatty acids. Supplement your diet with a good vitamin and mineral supplement powder from "Nutritech" to provide your body with quality vitamins and minerals.

Most importantly, make sure you take in your adequate supply of water on a daily basis. Keeping your body properly hydrated is a key in a healthy metabolism. Regulate your Leptin levels with the mentioned supplements that will help with the control of leptin. By sure to address any underlying hormonal problems that may be hindering your weight loss.

And most importantly – remember that you will lose the weight and keep it off permanently if you adhere what was mentioned in this book ! Great health to you and I wish you the best in your desire to lose weight.

Best of health to you !

Sincerely,
Tony Xhudo
If you would like to contact me or just have a quick question, feedback, etc...
cinncy63@ymail.com or please contact me on one of my blogs:
Muscle Health & Fitness Blog:
http://musclehealtandfitness.blog.com

Gaining Mass Muscle:
http://tonyxhudo.wordpress.com/

www.ingramcontent.com/pod-product-compliance
Lightning Source LLC
Chambersburg PA
CBHW082200290526
45794CB00008B/3365